Dash Diet: Lose Weight and Stay Fit

Dash Diet Cookbook for Beginners

Eleonore Barlow

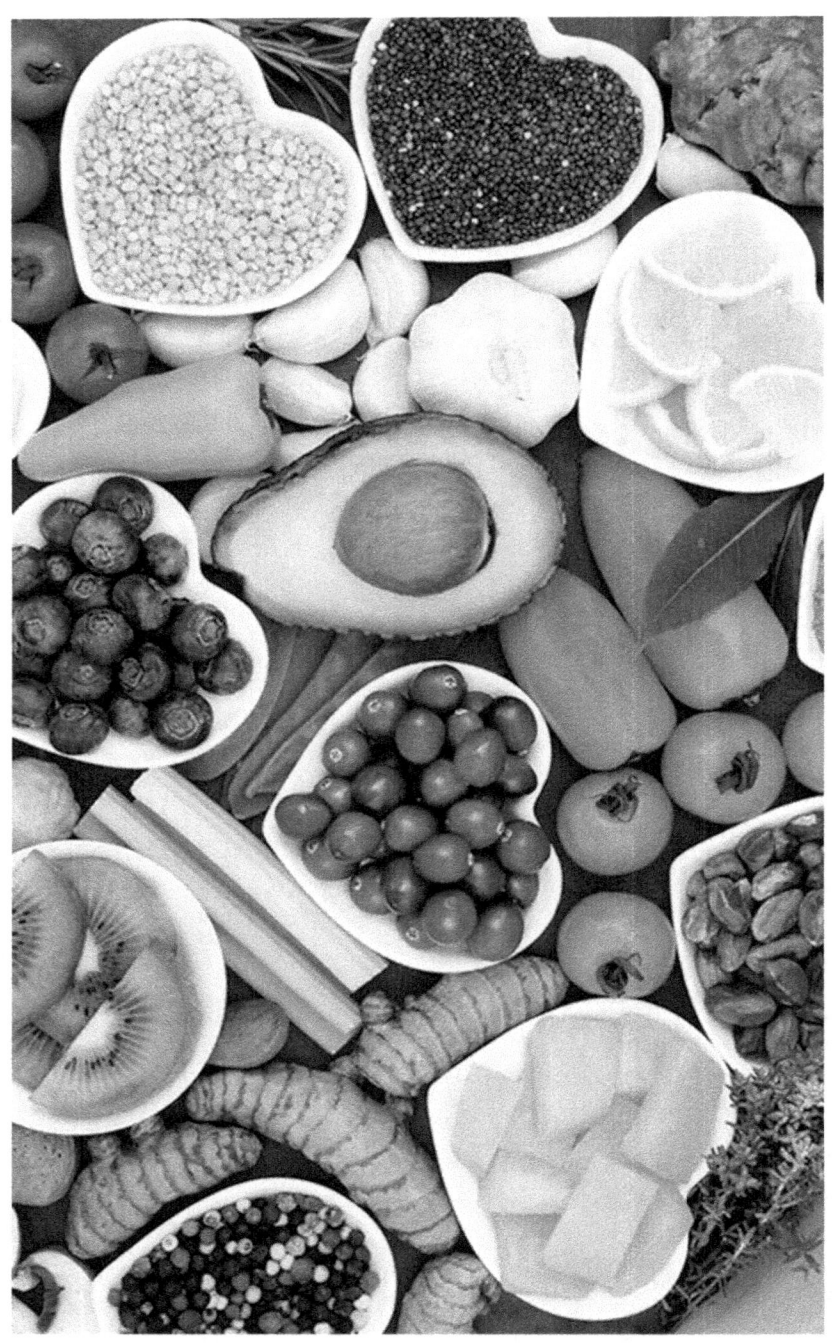

© Copyright 2021 - All rights reserved.

The content contained within this book may not be reproduced, duplicated or transmitted without direct written permission from the author or the publisher.
Under no circumstances will any blame or legal responsibility be held against the publisher, or author, for any damages, reparation, or monetary loss due to the information contained within this book. Either directly or indirectly.

Legal Notice:
This book is copyright protected. This book is only for personal use. You cannot amend, distribute, sell, use, quote or paraphrase any part, or the content within this book, without the consent of the author or publisher.

Disclaimer Notice:
Please note the information contained within this document is for educational and entertainment purposes only. All effort has been executed to present accurate, up to date, and reliable, complete information. No warranties of any kind are declared or implied. Readers acknowledge that the author is not engaging in the rendering of legal, financial, medical or professional advice. The content within this book has been derived from various sources. Please consult a licensed professional before attempting any techniques outlined in this book.
By reading this document, the reader agrees that under no circumstances is the author responsible for any losses, direct or indirect, which are incurred as a result of the use of information contained within this document, including, but not limited to, — errors, omissions, or inaccuracies.

Table of Contents

FANCY BANANA OATMEAL 6
TRADITIONAL FRITTATA 8
PEPPERONI OMELET 10
EGGY TOMATO SCRAMBLE 12
BREAKFAST FRUIT PIZZAS 14
PEANUT BUTTER OVERNIGHT OATS 16
WEDGE SALAD SKEWERS 18
HEARTY CHICKEN FRIED RICE 20
VEGGIE QUESADILLAS WITH CILANTRO YOGURT DIP 22
YOGURT WITH ALMONDS & HONEY 24
QUICK BUFFALO CHICKEN SALAD 25
ALL AMERICAN TUNA 27
PIMENTO CHEESE SANDWICH 28
HEARTY PORK BELLY CASSEROLE 29
APPLE PIE CRACKERS 31
PAPRIKA LAMB CHOPS 33
CHICKEN & GOAT CHEESE SKILLET 35
GREEN CURRY SALMON WITH GREEN BEANS 37
GREEK SALAD 39
FANCY GREEK ORZO SALAD 42
HOMELY TUSCAN TUNA SALAD 44
ASPARAGUS LOADED LOBSTER SALAD 46
TASTY YOGURT AND CUCUMBER SALAD 48
UNIQUE EGGPLANT SALAD 50
ZUCCHINI PESTO SALAD 52
PANKO-CRUSTED COD 54

GRILLED SALMON AND ASPARAGUS WITH LEMON BUTTER 56
PAN-ROASTED FISH FILLETS WITH HERB BUTTER............................ 59
CHILI MACADAMIA CRUSTED TILAPIA 61
BROILED WHITE SEA BASS... 63
GRILLED ASIAN SALMON... 65
PUMPKIN PIE FAT BOMBS 67
SENSATIONAL LEMONADE FAT BOMB... 69
SWEET ALMOND AND COCONUT FAT BOMBS 71
ALMOND AND TOMATO BALLS 73
AVOCADO TUNA BITES 75
MEDITERRANEAN POP CORN BITES.. 78
HEARTY BUTTERY WALNUTS... 80
FEISTY MANGO AND COCONUT SMOOTHIE 81
MEXICAN CHOCOLATE STAND-OFF 83
THE AWESOME CLEANSER 85
GENTLE TROPICAL PAPAYA SMOOTHIE 87
KALE AND APPLE SMOOTHIE 90
MANGO AND LIME GENEROUS SMOOTHIE 91
JUICY SUMMERTIME VEGGIES 93
CRAZY CARAMELIZED ONION 95
KIDNEY BEANS AND CILANTRO... 97
BROCCOLI CRUNCHIES 99
ULTIMATE BUFFALO CASHEWS..101
A GREEN BEAN MIXTURE 104

Fancy Banana Oatmeal

Serving: 4

Prep Time: 10 minutes

Cook Time: 10 minutes

Ingredients:

2 cups water

1 cup steel-cut oats

1 cup almond milk

¼ cup walnuts, chopped

2 tablespoons flaxseeds, ground

2 tablespoons chia seeds

2 bananas, peeled and mashed

1 teaspoon vanilla extract

1 teaspoon cinnamon powder

How To:

1. Add water, oats, almond milk, flaxseed, walnuts, chia seeds, vanilla, bananas, cinnamon to your Instant Pot and provides it a pleasant toss.

2. Lock the lid and cook on high for 10 minutes.

3. Release the pressure naturally and open the lid.

4. Divide the combination amongst bowls and serve.

5. Enjoy!

Nutrition (Per Serving)

Calories: 200

Fat: 4

Carbohydrates: 11g

Protein: 4g

Traditional Frittata

Serving: 6

Prep Time: 10 minutes

Cook Time: 5 minutes

Ingredients:

2 tablespoons almond milk

Just a pinch pepper

6 eggs, cracked and whisked

2 tablespoons parsley, chopped

1 tablespoon low-fat cheese, shredded

1 cup of water

How To:

1. Take a bowl and add the eggs, almond milk, pepper, cheese, and parsley. Whisk well.

2. Take a pan that might slot in your Instant Pot and grease with cooking spray.

3. Pour the egg mix into the pan.

4. Add a cup of water to your pot and place a steamer basket.

5. Add the pan within the basket.

6. Lock the lid and cook on high for five minutes.

7. Release the pressure naturally over 10 minutes.

8. Remove the lid and divide the frittata amongst serving plates.

9. Enjoy!

Nutrition (Per Serving)

Calories: 200

Fat: 4g

Carbohydrates: 17g

Protein: 6g

Pepperoni Omelet

Serving: 2

Prep Time: 5 minutes

Cook Time: 20 minutes

Ingredients:

3 eggs

7 pepperoni slices

1 teaspoon coconut cream

Salt and freshly ground black pepper, to taste 1 tablespoon butter

How To:

1. Take a bowl and whisk eggs with all the remaining ingredients in it.

2. Then take a skillet and warmth butter.

3. Pour quarter of the egg mixture into your skillet.

4. After that, cook for two minutes per side.

5. Repeat to use the whole batter.

6.   Serve warm and enjoy!

Nutrition (Per Serving)

Calories: 141

Fat: 11.5g

Carbohydrates: 0.6g

Protein: 8.9g

Eggy Tomato Scramble

Serving: 2

Prep Time: 10 minutes

Cook Time: 5 minutes

Ingredients:

2 whole eggs

½ cup fresh basil, chopped

2 tablespoons olive oil

½ teaspoon red pepper flakes, crushed

1 cup grape tomatoes, chopped

Salt and pepper to taste

How To:

1. Take a bowl and whisk in eggs, salt, pepper, red pepper flakes and blend well.

2. Add tomatoes, basil, and mix.

3. Take a skillet and place over medium-high heat.

4. Add the egg mixture and cook for five minutes until cooked and scrambled.

5. Enjoy!

Nutrition (Per Serving)

Calories: 130

Fat: 10g

Carbohydrates: 8g

Protein: 1.8g

Breakfast Fruit Pizzas

Ingredients

Two whole-wheat pita flatbreads

7 ounces Arla Original Cream Cheese

1-2 teaspoons honey

1/2 teaspoon pure vanilla extract

Three kiwi skin removed and sliced

1/2 cup sliced strawberries

1/2 cup blackberries

1/4 cup blueberries

Two raspberries for the center

Instructions

1. Preheat the oven to broil. Put the entire wheat pita flatbreads within the oven. Broil for 1 minute and switch over. Broilfor one minute more. you'll also toast the entire pita bread during a kitchen appliance. Set the dough aside to chill.

2. Take a bowl and blend the cheese, honey, and vanilla. Spread the cheese on the pita bread.

3.   Decorate the fruit on top of the cheese. dig slices and serve immediately.

4.   Note-you can use your favorite fruit. Bananas, peaches, pineapple, oranges, nectarines would even be good!

Peanut Butter Overnight Oats

Ingredients

Oats

Half of cup unsweetened plain almond milk (or sub other dairy-free milk, such as coconut, soy, or hemp!) 3/4 Tbsp of chia seed

2 Tbsp of natural salted peanut butter or almond butter (creamy or crunchy // or sub other nut or seed butter)

1 Tbsp of maple syrup (or sub coconut sugar, natural brown sugar, or stevia to taste) half of cup gluten-loose rolled oats (rolled oats are best, vs. Steel-cut or quick-cooking) Toppings optional

Sliced banana, strawberries, or raspberries Flaxseed meal or additional chia seed Granola

Instructions

1. Take a little bowl with a lid, add almond milk, chia seeds, spread, and syrup (or every other sweetener) and stir with a spoon to mix. The spread doesn't got to be alright blended with the almond milk (doing so leaves swirls of spread to enjoy the next day).

2. Add oats and stir a couple of extra times. Then depress with a spoon to form sure all oats were moistened and areimmersed in almond milk.

3. Cover tightly with a lid or seal and set within the fridge overnight (or for a minimum of 6 hours) to place/soak.

4. the next day, open and knowledge as is or garnish with preferred toppings.

5. Overnight oats will preserve within the refrigerator for 2-three days, though high-quality within the primary 12-24 hours in our experience. Not freezer friendly.

Nutrition

Calories: 452, Fat: 22.8g, Saturated fat: 4.1g, Sodium: 229mgPotassium:479mgCarbohydrates: 51.7g Fiber: 8.3gSugar: 15.8g Protein: 14.6g

Wedge Salad Skewers

Ingredients

One head of iceberg lettuce (cut into wedge pieces)

Four Roma tomatoes cut in half

One red onion (cut into 1-inch pieces)

Two avocados cut into 1-inch pieces

Five slices of bacon cooked and cut into thirds

One cucumber (sliced (peeled or unpeeled))

Eight wooden skewers

Two green onions (diced)

1 5 oz container blue cheese crumbles One bottle blue cheese dressing

Instructions

1.   One skewer at a time adds an iceberg wedge, tomato, onion, avocado, two pieces of bacon, every other iceberg wedge, and then cucumber.

2. Continue till all skewers have been made, then garnish with crumbled blue cheese, blue cheese dressing, and diced leafy green onions.

Nutrition

Calories: 238kcal, Fat: 19g, Saturated fat: 6gCholesterol: 25mg Sodium: 401mgPotassium: 573mgCarbohydrates: 10g Fiber: 5g Sugar: 3gProtein: 8gVitamin A: 890%Vitamin C: 13.9%Calcium: 144%Iron: 0.9%

Hearty Chicken Fried Rice

Serving: 4

Prep Time: 10 minutes

Cook Time: 12 minutes

Ingredients:

1 teaspoon olive oil

4 large egg whites

1 onion, chopped

2 garlic cloves, minced

12 ounces skinless chicken breasts, boneless, cut into ½ inch cubes

½ cup carrots, chopped

½ cup frozen green peas

2 cups long grain brown rice, cooked

3 tablespoons soy sauce, low sodium

How To:

1. Coat skillet with oil, place it over medium-high heat.
2. Add egg whites and cook until scrambled.
3. Sauté onion, garlic and chicken breasts for six minutes.
4. Add carrots, peas and keep cooking for 3 minutes.
5. Stir in rice, season with soy.
6. Add cooked egg whites, stir for 3 minutes.
7. Enjoy!

Nutrition (Per Serving)

Calories: 353

Fat: 11g

Carbohydrates: 30g

Protein: 23g

Veggie Quesadillas with Cilantro Yogurt Dip

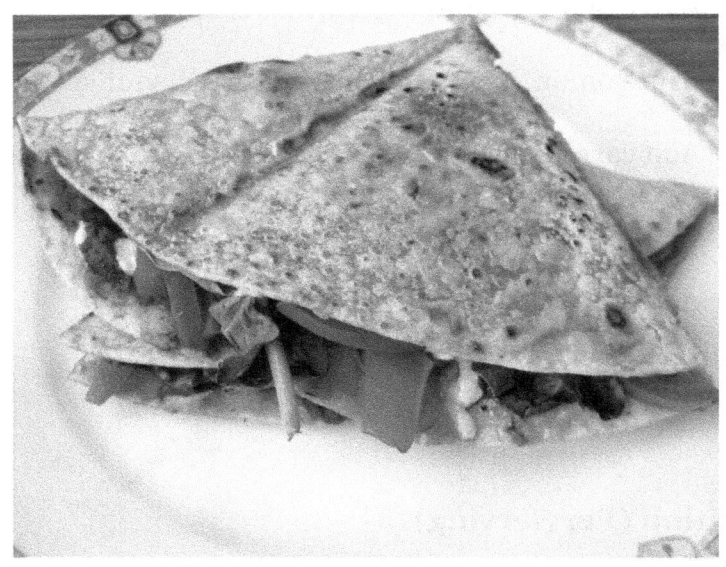

Ingredients

1 cup beans, black or pinto

2 Tablespoons cilantro, chopped

½ bell pepper, finely chopped

½ cup corn kernels

1 cup low-fat shredded cheese

Six soft corn tortillas

One medium carrot, shredded

½ jalapeno pepper, finely minced (optional)

CILANTRO YOGURT DIP

1 cup plain nonfat yogurt

2 Tablespoons cilantro, finely chopped

Juice from ½ of a lime

Instructions

1. Preheat large skillet over low heat.

2. Line up three tortillas. Spread cheese, corn, beans, cilantro, shredded carrots, and peppers over the tortillas.

3. Cover all sides with a 2nd tortilla.

4. Place a tortilla on a dry plate and warmth until cheese is melted and tortilla is slightly golden after 3 minutes.

5. Flip and cook another side until golden, about 1 minute.

6. Inside a small bowl, mix the nonfat yogurt, cilantro, and juice.

7. Cut each quesadilla into four wedges (12 wedges total) and serve three wedges per person with about ¼ cup of the dip.

8. Refrigerate leftovers within 2 hours.

Yogurt with Almonds & Honey

Ingredients

Non-fat greek yoghurt-Nonfat, plain-16 oz-453 grams

Almonds-Nuts, raw-1/4 cup, whole-35.8 grams

Honey-2 tsp-14.1 grams

Directions

Rough-chop almonds and blend into yogurt and honey. Enjoy!

Nutrition

Calories 517 Carbs 36g Fat 20g Protein 54g Fiber 5g Net carbs 31g Sodium 164mg Cholesterol 23mg

Quick Buffalo Chicken Salad

Ingredients

Pepper or hot sauce-Ready-to-serve-4 tbsp-57.6 grams

Canned chicken-No broth-1 cup-205 grams

Spinach-Raw-2 cup-60 grams

Tomatoes-Green, raw-Two medium-246 grams

Directions

Mix hot sauce with chicken. Spread spinach and tomatoes on the top. Toss together and enjoy it!

Nutrition

Calorie 456 Carbs 18g Fat 18g Protein 57g Fiber 4g Net carbs 13g Sodium 2590mg Cholesterol 103mg

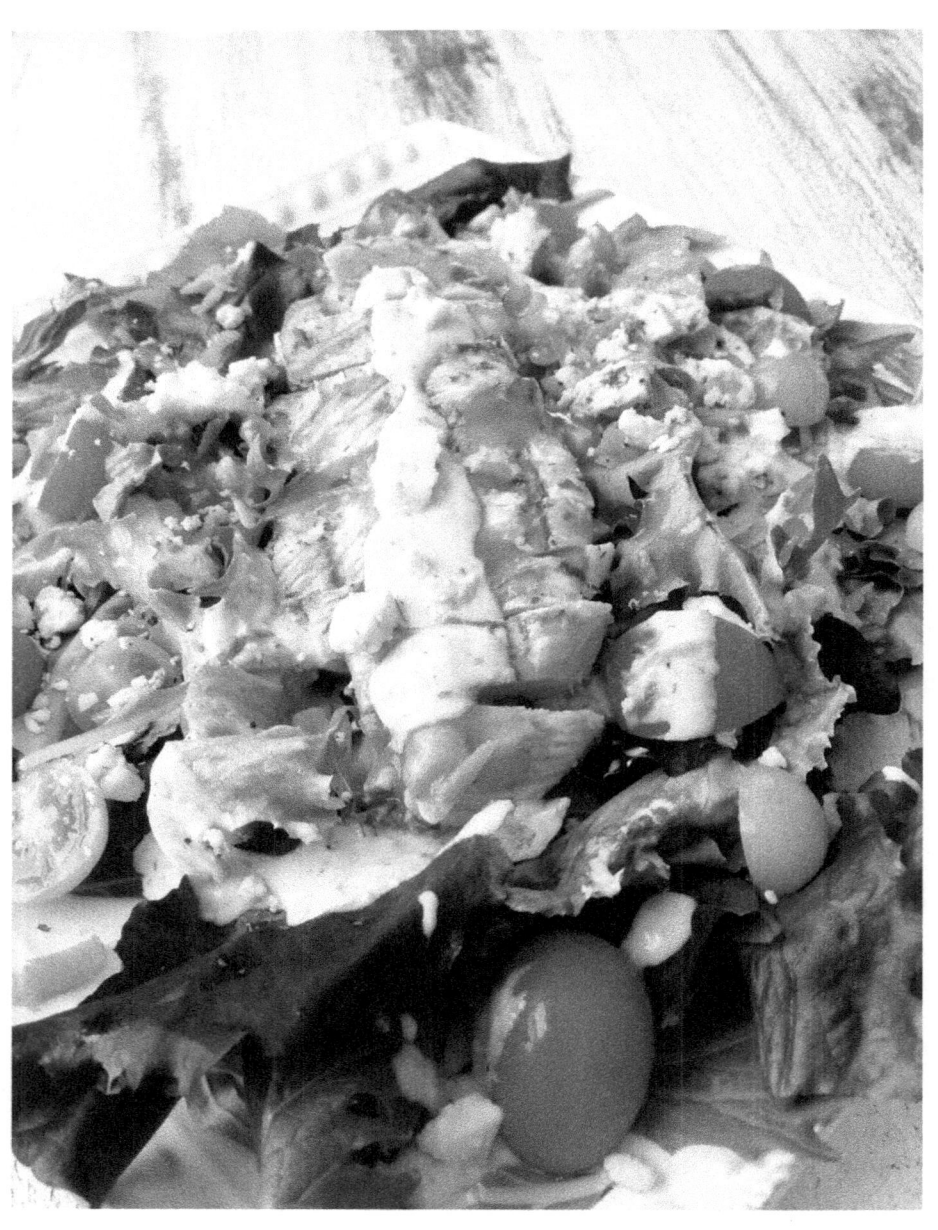

All American Tuna

Ingredients

Tuna-Fish, light, canned in water, drained solids-Two can-330 grams

Light mayonnaise-Salad dressing, light-2 tbsp-30 grams Celery-Cooked, boiled, drained, without a salt-1/4 cup, diced-37.5 grams

Pickles-Cucumber, dill or kosher dill-One large (4" long)-135 grams

Wheat bread-Two slice-50 grams

Directions

1. Mix all ingredients in a bowl.
2. Serve with bread.

Nutrition

Calories 512 Carbs 32g Fat 12g Protein 71g Fiber 4g Net carbs 28g Sodium 2443mg Cholesterol 124mg

Pimento Cheese Sandwich

Ingredients

Pimento cheese-Pasteurized process-2 oz-56.7 grams Multi-grain bread-Four slices regular-104 grams

Directions

1. Spread the pimento cheese over the bread.
2. Then, a slice of bread to form a sandwich. Enjoy!

Nutrition

Calories 488 Carbs 46g Fat 22g Protein 26g Fiber 8g Net carbs 38g Sodium 915mg Cholesterol 53mg

Hearty Pork Belly Casserole

Serving: 4

Prep Time: 5 minutes

Cook Time: 25 minutes

Ingredients:

8 pork belly slices, cut into small pieces

3 large onions, chopped

4 tablespoons lemon

Juice of 1 lemon

Seasoning as you needed

How To:

1.   Take an outsized autoclave and place it over medium heat.

2.   Add onions and sweat them for five minutes.

3.   Add side of pork slices and cook until the meat browns and onions become golden.

4. Cover with water and add honey, lemon peel, sunflower seeds, pepper, and shut the pressure seal.

5. Pressure cook for 40 minutes.

6. Serve and luxuriate in with a garnish of fresh chopped parsley if you favor.

Nutrition (Per Serving)

Calories: 753

Fat: 41g

Carbohydrates: 68g

Protein: 30g

Apple Pie Crackers

Serving: 100 crackers

Prep Time: 10 minutes

Cooking Time: 120 minutes

Ingredients:

2 tablespoons + 2 teaspoons avocado oil

1 medium Granny Smith apple, roughly chopped ¼ cup Erythritol

1/4 cup sunflower seeds, ground

1 ¾ cups roughly ground flax seeds

1/8 teaspoon Ground cloves

1/8 teaspoon ground cardamom

3 tablespoons nutmeg

¼ teaspoon ground ginger

How To:

1. Pre-heat your oven to 225 degrees F.

2. Line two baking sheets with parchment paper and keep them on the side.

3. Add oil, apple, Erythritol to a bowl and blend.

4. Transfer to kitchen appliance and add remaining ingredients, process until combined.

5. Transfer batter to baking sheets, spread evenly and dig crackers.

6. Bake for 1 hour, flip and bake for an additional hour.

7. allow them to cool and serve.

8. Enjoy!

Nutrition (Per Serving)

Total Carbs: 0.9g (%)

Fiber: 0.5g

Protein: 0.4g (%)

Fat: 2.1g (%)

Paprika Lamb Chops

Serving: 4

Prep Time: 10 minutes

Cook Time: 15 minutes

Ingredients:

1 lamb rack, cut into chops pepper to taste 1 tablespoon paprika

1/2 cup cumin powder

1/2 teaspoon chili powder

How To:

1. Take a bowl and add paprika, cumin, chili, pepper, and stir.
2. Add lamb chops and rub the mixture.
3. Heat grill over medium-temperature and add lamb chops, cook for five minutes.
4. Flip and cook for five minutes more, flip again.
5. Cook for two minutes, flip and cook for two minutes more.

6.   Serve and enjoy!

Nutrition (Per Serving)

Calories: 200

Fat: 5g

Carbohydrates: 4g

Protein: 8g

Chicken & Goat Cheese Skillet

Ingredients

1/2 pound of boneless skinless chicken breasts, cut into 1-inch pieces

1/4 teaspoon salt

1/8 teaspoon pepper

Two teaspoons olive oil

1 cup sliced fresh asparagus (1-inch pieces)

One garlic clove, minced

Three plum tomatoes, chopped

Three tablespoons 2% milk

Two tablespoons herbed fresh goat cheese, crumbled Hot cooked rice or pasta

Additional goat cheese, optional

Directions

1.	Toss chicken with salt and pepper. Heat oil at medium heat; saute chicken until not pink, 4-6 minutes.Remove from pan; keep warm.

2. Add asparagus to skillet; cook and blend at medium-high heat 1 minute. Add garlic; cook and stir 30 seconds. Stirin tomatoes, milk, and two tablespoons cheese; cook, covered, over medium heat until cheese begins to melt, 2-3 minutes. Stir in chicken. Serve with rice. If desired, top with additional cheese.

Nutrition

251 calories, 11g fat, 74mg cholesterol, 447mg sodium, 8g carbohydrate (5g sugars, 3g fiber), 29g protein. Diabetic Exchanges: 4 lean meat, two fat, one vegetable.

Green Curry Salmon with Green Beans

Ingredients

Four salmon fillets (4 ounces each)

1 cup light coconut milk

Two tablespoons green curry paste

1 cup uncooked instant brown rice

1 cup reduced-sodium chicken broth

1/8 teaspoon pepper

3/4-pound fresh green beans, trimmed

One teaspoon sesame oil

One teaspoon sesame seeds, toasted

Lime wedges

Directions

1. Preheat oven to 400°. Place salmon in an 8-in. Square baking dish. Mix together coconut milk and curry paste; pour over salmon. Bake, uncovered, till fish simply starts offevolved to flake effortlessly with a fork, 15-20 minutes.

2.	Meanwhile, during a small saucepan, integrate rice, broth and pepper; convey to a boil. Reduce warmth; simmer, covered, 5 minutes. Remove from heat; let stand five minutes.

3.	In a big saucepan, area steamer basket over 1 in. Of water. Place inexperienced beans inside the basket; convey water to a boil. Reduce heat to take care of a simmer; steam, covered, till beans are crisp-tender, 7-10 minutes. Toss with vegetable oil and sesame seeds.

4.	Serve salmon with rice, beans and lime wedges. Spoon coconut sauce over the salmon.

Nutrition Facts

366 calories, 17g fat (5g saturated fat), 57mg cholesterol, 340mg sodium, 29g carbohydrate (5g sugars, 4g fibre), 24g protein.

Greek Salad

Serving: 4

Prep Time: 6 minutes

Cook Time: Nil

Ingredients:

2 cucumbers, diced

2 tomatoes, sliced

1 green lettuce, cut into thin strips

2 red bell peppers, cut

½ cup black olives pitted

3 ½ ounces feta cheese, cut

1 red onion, sliced

2 tablespoons olive oil

2 tablespoons lemon juice

Sunflower seeds and pepper to taste

Direction

1. Dice cucumbers and slice up the tomatoes.

2. Tear the lettuce and cut it into thin strips.

3. De-seed and cut the peppers into strips.

4. Take a salad bowl and mix in all the listed vegetables, add olives and feta cheese (cut into cubes).

5. Take a small cup and mix in olive oil and lemon juice, season with sunflower seeds and pepper.

6. Pour mixture into the salad and toss well, enjoy!

Nutrition (Per Serving)

Calories: 132

Fat: 4g

Carbohydrates: 3g

Protein: 5g

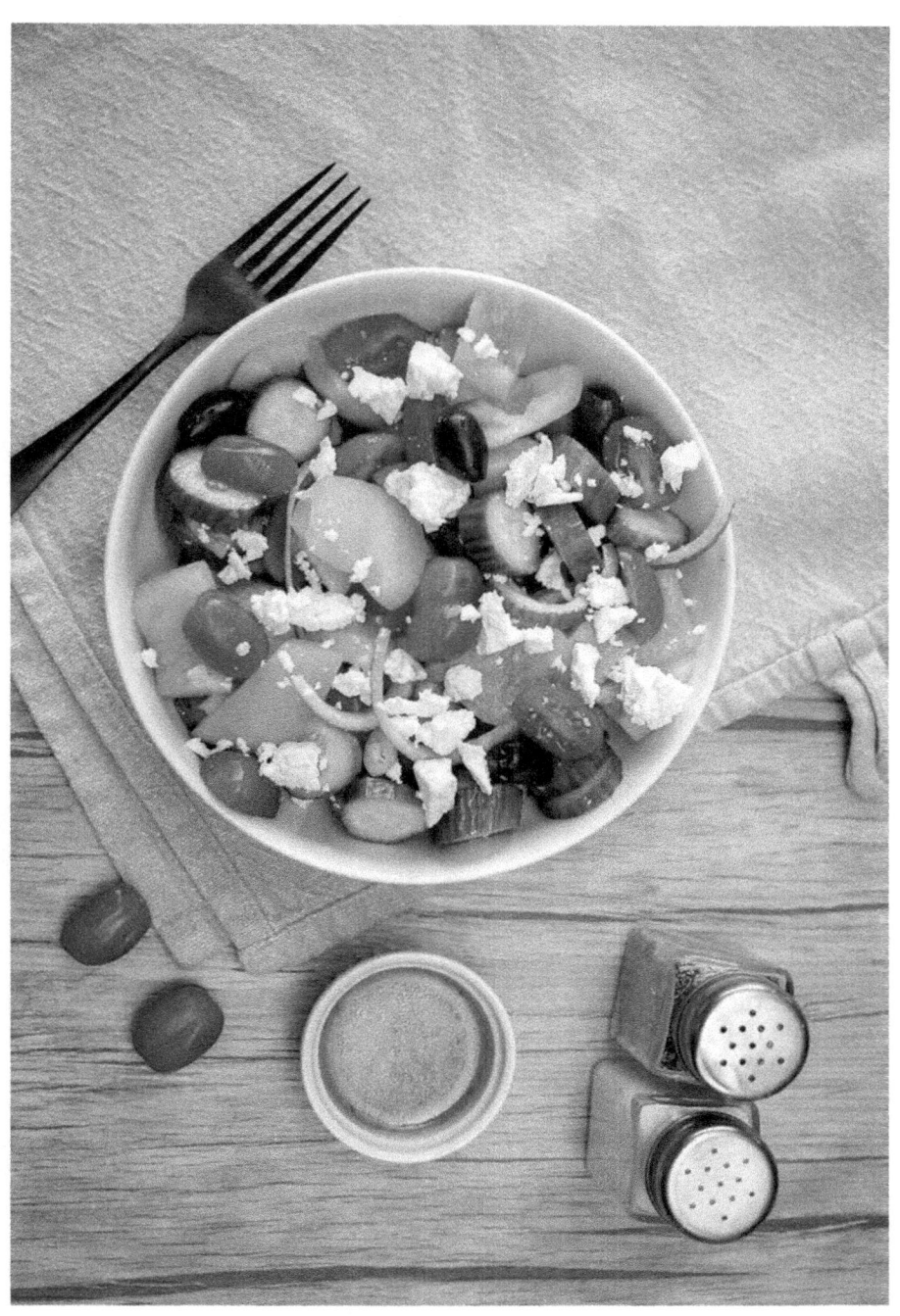

Fancy Greek Orzo Salad

Serving: 4

Prep Time: 5 minutes and 24 hours chill time

Cook Time: 10 minutes

Ingredients:

1 cup orzo pasta, uncooked

½ cup fresh parsley, minced

6 teaspoons olive oil

1 onion, chopped

1 ½ teaspoons oregano

How To:

1. Cook the orzo and drain them.
2. Add to a serving dish.
3. Add 2 teaspoons of oil.
4. Take another dish and add parsley, onion, remaining oil and oregano.

5. Season with sunflower seeds, pepper according to your taste.

6. Pour the mixture over the orzo and let it chill for 24 hours.

7. Serve and enjoy at lunch!

Nutrition (Per Serving)

Calories: 399

Fat: 12g

Carbohydrates: 55g

Protein:16g

Homely Tuscan Tuna Salad

Serving: 4

Prep Time: 5-10 minutes

Cook Time: Nil

Ingredients:

15 ounces small white beans

6 ounces drained chunks of light tuna

cherry tomatoes, quartered

4 scallions, trimmed and sliced

2 tablespoons lemon juice

How To:

Add all of the listed ingredients to a bowl and gently stir.

Season with sunflower seeds and pepper accordingly, enjoy!

Nutrition (Per Serving)

Calories: 322

Fat: 8g

Carbohydrates: 32g

Protein:30g

Asparagus Loaded Lobster Salad

Serving: 4

Prep Time: 10 minutes

Cook Time: Nil

Ingredients:

8 ounces lobster, cooked and chopped

3 ½ cups asparagus, chopped and steamed

2 tablespoons lemon juice

4 teaspoons extra virgin olive oil

¼ teaspoon kosher sunflower seeds

Pepper

½ cup cherry tomatoes halved

1 basil leaf, chopped

2 tablespoons red onion, diced

How To:

1.   Whisk in lemon juice, sunflower seeds, pepper in a bowl and mix with oil.

2.   Take a bowl and add the rest of the ingredients.

3.   Toss well and pour dressing on top.

Serve and enjoy!

Nutrition (Per Serving)

Calories: 247

Fat: 10g

Carbohydrates: 14g

Protein: 27g

Tasty Yogurt and Cucumber Salad

Serving: 4

Prep Time: 10 minutes

Cook Time: Nil

Ingredients:

5-6 small cucumbers, peeled and diced

1 (8 ounces) container plain Greek yogurt

2 garlic cloves, minced

1 tablespoon fresh mint, minced

Sea sunflower seeds and fresh black pepper

How To:

Take a large bowl and add cucumbers, garlic, yogurt, mint.

Season with sunflower seeds and pepper.

Refrigerate the salad for 1 hour and serve.

Enjoy!

Nutrition (Per Serving)

Calories: 74

Fat: 0.7g

Carbohydrates: 16g

Protein: 2g

Unique Eggplant Salad

Serving: 3

Prep Time: 10 minutes

Cook Time: 30 minutes

Ingredients:

2 eggplants, peeled and sliced

2 garlic cloves

2 green bell pepper, sliced, seeds removed ½ cup fresh parsley

½ cup mayonnaise, low fat, low sodium Sunflower seeds and black pepper

How To:

1. Preheat your oven to 480 degrees F.

2. Take a baking pan and add eggplant, bell peppers and season with black [MOU15][F16]pepper to it.

3. Bake for about 30 minutes.

4. Flip the vegetables after 20 minutes.

5. Then, take a bowl, add baked vegetables and all the remaining ingredients.

6. Mix well.

7. Serve and enjoy!

Nutrition (Per Serving)

Calories: 196

Fat: 108.g

Carbohydrates: 13.4g

Protein: 14.6g

Zucchini Pesto Salad

Serving: 4

Prep Time: 10 minutes

Cook Time: 10 minutes

Ingredients:

2 cups spiral pasta

2 zucchini, sliced and halved

4 tomatoes, cut

1 cup white mushrooms, cut

1 small red onion, chopped

2 tablespoons fresh basil leaves, chopped

2 tablespoons sunflower oil

1 tablespoon lemon juice

Pepper and sunflower seeds to taste

How To:

1. Cook the pasta according to the package instructions, drain and rinse under cold water.

2. Take a large bowl and add zucchini, tomatoes, mushrooms, onion, and pasta.

3. Mix well,

4. In a food processor, add oil, lemon juice, basil, blue cheese, black, and process well.

5. Pour the mixture over the salad and toss well.

6. Serve and enjoy!

Nutrition (Per Serving)

Calories: 301

Fat: 25g

Net Carbohydrates: 7g

Protein: 10g

Panko-Crusted Cod

Prep time: 10 minutes

Cook time: 15 minutes

Servings: 2

Ingredients

Panko-style breadcrumbs – ¼ cup Garlic - 1 clove, minced Extra-virgin olive oil – 1 Tbsp. Nonfat Greek yogurt – 3 Tbsp. Mayonnaise – 1 Tbsp.

Lemon juice – 1 ½ tsp.

Tarragon – ½ tsp.

Pinch of salt

Cod – 10 ounces, cut into two portions

Method

1. Preheat the oven to 425F.
2. Coat a baking pan with cooking spray.
3. In a bowl, combine olive oil, garlic, and breadcrumbs.
4. In another bowl, combine lemon juice, mayonnaise, yogurt, tarragon, and salt.
5. Place fish in the baking pan. Top each piece with one-half yogurt mixture then 1/3 breadcrumb mixture.
6. Bake in the oven for 15 minutes.

7. Serve.

Nutritional Facts Per Serving

Calories: 225

Fat: 10g

Carb: 13g

Protein: 18g

Sodium 270mg

Grilled Salmon and Asparagus with Lemon Butter

Prep time: 10 minutes

Cook time: 20 minutes

Servings: 4

Ingredients

Salmon – 1 ¼ pound, cut into 4 portions Asparagus – 2 bunches, ends trimmed Olive oil cooking spray Salt – ½ tsp. Freshly ground black pepper – ¼ tsp. Garlic powder – ¼ tsp. Olive oil – 1 Tbsp.

Butter – 1 Tbsp.

Lemon juice – 3 Tbsp.

Method

1. On a baking sheet, place the salmon and asparagus. Spray lightly with cooking spray. Season with salt, pepper, and garlic powder.
2. Grease and preheat grill. Place salmon and asparagus on it.
3. Grill total 6 minutes, 3 minutes per side, or until opaque, turning once.
4. Grill the asparagus for 5 to 7 minutes, or until tender, turning occasionally.

5. In a bowl, place butter, olive oil, and lemon juice. Microwave to melt.

6. Drizzle fish with this mixture.

7. Serve.

Nutritional Facts Per Serving

Calories: 190

Fat: 8g

Carb: 6g

Protein: 24g

Sodium 445mg

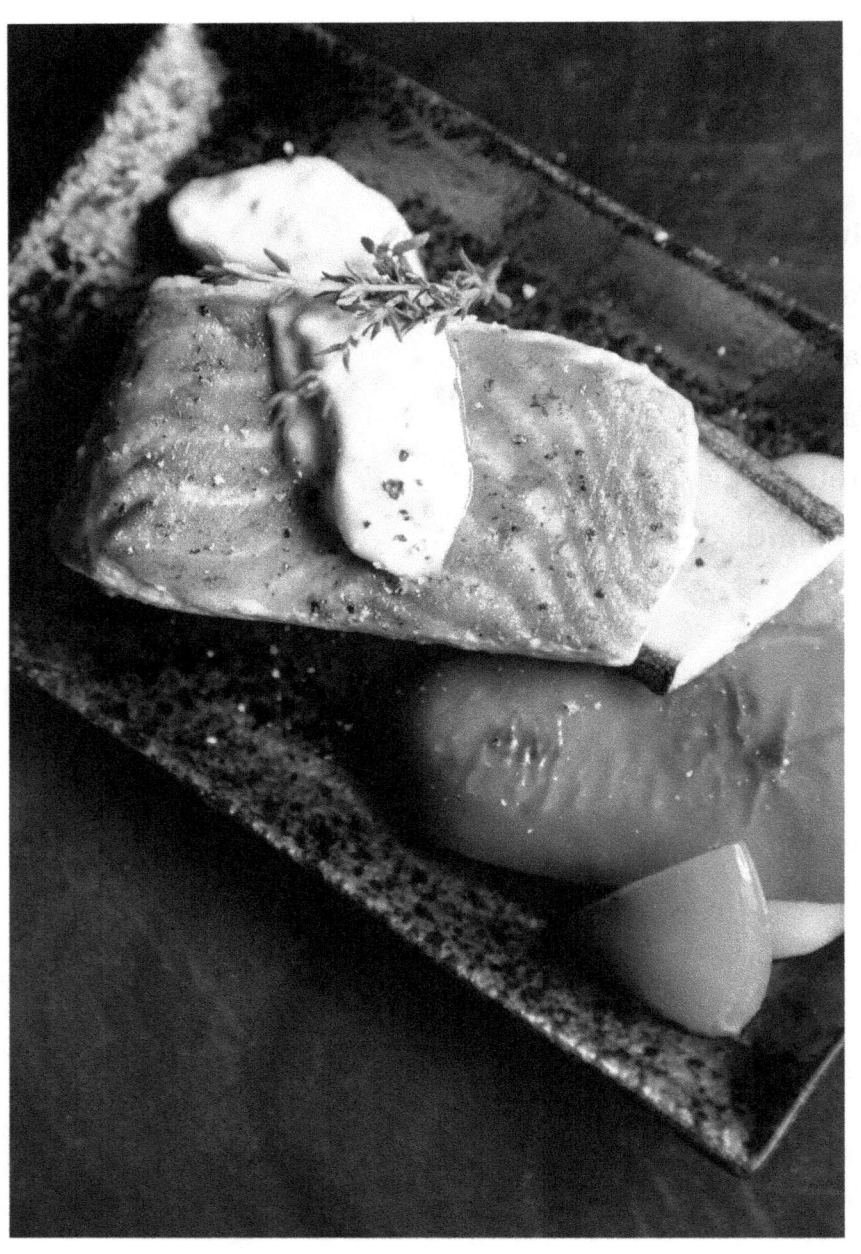

Pan-Roasted Fish Fillets with Herb Butter

Prep time: 10 minutes

Cook time: 5 minutes

Servings: 2

Ingredients

Fish fillets – 2 (5-ounce each) ½ to 1-inch-thick Salt – ¼ tsp.

Ground black pepper Olive oil – 3 Tbsp.

Unsalted butter -1 Tbsp. divided

Fresh thyme – 2 sprigs

Chopped flat-leaf parsley - 1 Tbsp. Lemon wedges

Method

1. Rub the fish with pepper and salt.

2. Heat oil in a skillet.

3. Place fillets and cook until around the edges, about 2 to 3 minutes. Then flip the fillets and add the butter and thyme to the pan.

4. Baste the fish with melted butter until golden all over, about 2 minutes.

5. Serve with chopped parsley and lemon wedges.

Nutritional Facts Per Serving

Calories: 369

Fat: 26.9g

Carb: 1g

Protein: 30.5g

Sodium 62mg

Chili Macadamia Crusted Tilapia

Prep time: 20 minutes

Cook time: 7 minutes

Servings: 4

Ingredients

Tilapia fillets – 4

Macadamia nuts – ½ cup, chopped coarsely

Whole wheat panko crumbs – ½ cup Chili powder – 1 tsp.

Cayenne pepper – ¼ tsp.

Paprika – ¼ tsp.

Salt – ¼ tsp.

Pepper – ¼ tsp.

Egg – 1

Olive oil – 3 Tbsp.

Method

1. In a bowl, combine panko crumbs, nuts, chili powder, cayenne pepper, paprika, salt, and pepper.

2. Whisk egg in another bowl and set aside.

3. Heat the olive oil in a skillet.

4. Dredge each tilapia fillet in the egg and then coat it in the macadamia-spice-panko mixture.

5. Cook fillets until browned and cooked through, about 3 minutes on each side.

6. Serve.

Nutritional Facts Per Serving

Calories: 351

Fat: 26.5g

Carb: 5.7g

Protein: 25.7g

Sodium 234mg

Broiled White Sea Bass

Prep time: 5 minutes

Cook time: 10 minutes

Servings: 2

Ingredients

White sea bass fillets – 2, each 4 ounces Lemon juice – 1 Tbsp. Garlic – 1 tsp. minced

Salt-free herb seasoning blend – ¼ tsp. Ground black pepper to taste

Method

1. Heat the broiler (grill).

2. Place the rack very close (4 inches) to the heat source.

3. Place the fillets in a greased baking pan.

4. Sprinkle the fillets with herbed seasoning, garlic, lemon juice, and pepper.

5. Broil (grill) until opaque throughout, about 8 to 10 minutes

6. Serve.

Nutritional Facts Per Serving

Calories: 102

Fat: 2g

Carb: 1g

Protein: 21g

Sodium 77mg

Grilled Asian Salmon

Prep time: 1 hour

Cook time: 10 minutes

Servings: 4

Ingredients

Sesame oil – 1 Tbsp.

Homemade soy sauce – 1 Tbsp.

Fresh ginger – 1 Tbsp. minced Rice wine vinegar – 1 Tbsp.

Salmon fillets – 4, each 4 ounces

Method

1. Combine vinegar, ginger, soy sauce, and sesame oil in a dish.

2. Add salmon and coat well. Marinate for 1 hour, turning occasionally (in the refrigerator).

3. Grease a grill and heat over medium heat.

4. Grill the salmon on 5 minutes per side or until almost opaque.

5. Serve.

Nutritional Facts Per Serving

Calories: 185

Fat: 9g

Carb: 1g

Protein: 26g

Sodium 113mg

Pumpkin Pie Fat Bombs

Serving: 12

Prep Time: 35 minutes

Cooking Time: 5 minutes

Freeze Time: 3 hours

Ingredients:

2 tablespoons coconut oil

1/3 cup pumpkin puree

1/3 cup almond oil

¼ cup almond oil

3 ounces sugar-free dark chocolate

1 ½ teaspoons pumpkin pie spice mix Stevia to taste

How To:

1. Melt almond oil and dark chocolate over a double boiler.
2. Take this mixture and layer the bottom of 12 muffin cups.
3. Freeze until the crust has set.

4. Meanwhile, take a saucepan and combine the rest of the ingredients.

5. Put the saucepan on low heat.

6. Heat until softened and mix well.

7. Pour this over the initial chocolate mixture.

8. Let it chill for at least 1 hour.

Nutrition (Per Serving)

Total Carbs: 3g

Fiber: 1g

Protein: 3g

Fat: 13g

Calories: 124

Sensational Lemonade Fat Bomb

Serving: 2

Prep Time: 2 hours

Cook Time: Nil

Ingredients:

½ lemon

4 ounces cream cheese

2 ounces almond butter

Salt to taste

2 teaspoons natural sweetener

How To:

1. Take a fine grater and zest lemon.

2. Squeeze lemon juice into bowl with zest.

3. Add butter, cream cheese in a bowl and add zest, juice, salt, sweetener.

4. Mix well using a hand mixer until smooth.

5. Spoon mixture into molds and let them freeze for 2 hours.

6. Serve and enjoy!

Nutrition (Per Serving)

Calories: 404

Fat: 43g

Carbohydrates: 4g

Protein: 4g

Sweet Almond and Coconut Fat Bombs

Serving: 6

Prep Time: 10 minutes

Cooking Time: / Freeze Time: 20 minutes

Ingredients:

¼ cup melted coconut oil

9 ½ tablespoons almond butter

90 drops liquid stevia

3 tablespoons cocoa

9 tablespoons melted butter, salted

How To:

1. Take a bowl and add all of the listed ingredients.

2. Mix them well.

3. Pour scant 2 tablespoons of the mixture into as many muffin molds as you like.

4. Chill for 20 minutes and pop them out.

5. Serve and enjoy!

Nutrition (Per Serving)

Total Carbs: 2g

Fiber: 0g

Protein: 2.53g

Fat: 14g

Almond and Tomato Balls

Serving: 6

Prep Time: 10 minutes

Cooking Time: / Freeze Time: 20 minutes

Ingredients:

1/3 cup pistachios, de-shelled

10 ounces cream cheese

1/3 cup sun dried tomatoes, diced

How To:

1. Chop pistachios into small pieces.
2. Add cream cheese, tomatoes in a bowl and mix well.
3. Chill for 15-20 minutes and turn into balls.
4. Roll into pistachios.
5. Serve and enjoy!

Nutrition (Per Serving)

Carb: 183

Fat: 18g

Carb: 5g

Protein: 5g

Avocado Tuna Bites

Serving: 4

Prep Time: 10 minutes

Cook Time: nil

Ingredients:

1/3 cup coconut oil

1 avocado, cut into cubes

10 ounces canned tuna, drained

¼ cup parmesan cheese, grated

¼ teaspoon garlic powder

1/4 teaspoon onion powder

1/3 cup almond flour

¼ teaspoon pepper

¼ cup low fat mayonnaise Pepper as needed

How To:

1. Take a bowl and add tuna, mayo, flour, parmesan, spices and mix well.

2. Fold in avocado and make 12 balls out of the mixture.

3. Melt coconut oil in pan and cook over medium heat, until all sides are golden.

4. Serve and enjoy!

Nutrition (Per Serving)

Calories: 185

Fat: 18g

Carbohydrates: 1g

Protein: 5g

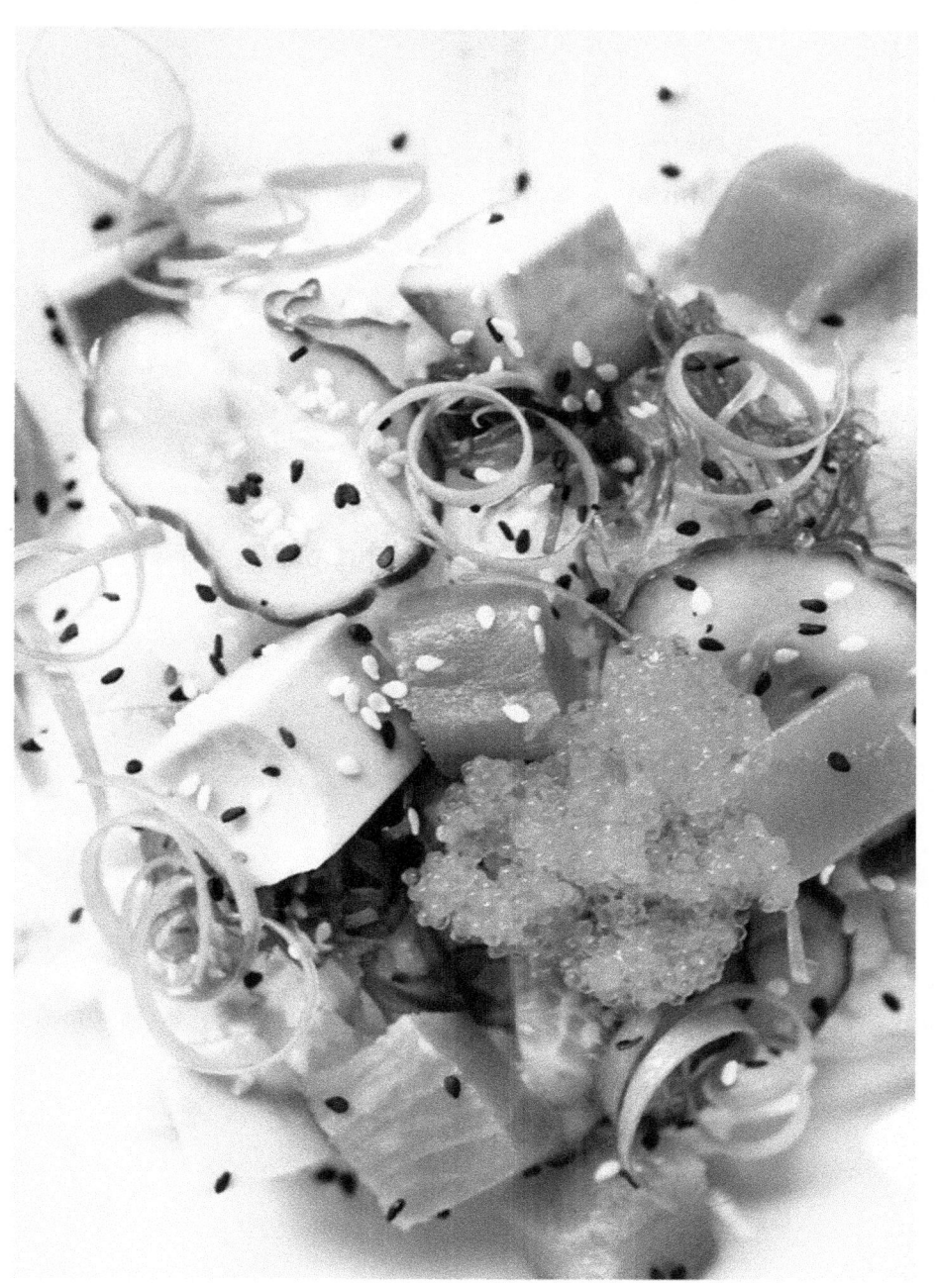

Mediterranean Pop Corn Bites

Serving: 4

Prep Time: 5 minutes + 20 minutes chill time

Cook Time: 2-3 minutes

Ingredients:

3 cups Medjool dates, chopped

12 ounces brewed coffee 1 cup pecan, chopped ½ cup coconut, shredded ½ cup cocoa powder

How To:

1. Soak dates in warm coffee for 5 minutes.

2. Remove dates from coffee and mash them, making a fine smooth mixture.

3. Stir in remaining ingredients (except cocoa powder) and form small balls out of the mixture.

4. Coat with cocoa powder, serve and enjoy!

Nutrition (Per Serving)

Calories: 265

Fat: 12g

Carbohydrates: 43g

Protein 3g

Hearty Buttery Walnuts

Serving: 4

Prep Time: 10 minutes

Cook Time: nil

Ingredients:

4 walnut halves

½ tablespoon almond butter

How To:

1. Spread butter over two walnut halves.
2. Top with other halves.
3. Serve and enjoy!

Nutrition (Per Serving)

Calories: 90

Fat: 10g

Carbohydrates: 0g

Protein: 1g

Feisty Mango and Coconut Smoothie

Serving: 2

Prep Time: 5 minutes

Ingredients:

1 teaspoon spirulina

1 cup frozen mango

1 cup unsweetened coconut milk

½ cup spinach

How To:

1. Cut mangoes and dice them.

2. Add mango, cup of unsweetened coconut milk, teaspoon of Spirulina and spinach to the blender.

3. Blend on low to medium until smooth.

4. Check the texture and serve chilled!

Nutrition (Per Serving)

Calories: 200

Fat: 10g

Carbohydrates: 14g

Protein 2g

Mexican Chocolate Stand-Off

Serving: 2

Prep Time: 5 minutes

Ingredients:

2 bananas

1 tablespoon hemp seeds

1 bag frozen blueberries

½ teaspoon liquid stevia

Pure water

2 teaspoons raw chocolate

1 teaspoon raw carob powder

½ teaspoon green powder

½ teaspoon cinnamon powder

Pinch of cayenne pepper

How To:

1. Add all the listed ingredients to your blender.
2. Blend until smooth.

3. Add a few ice cubes and serve the smoothie.

4. Enjoy!

Nutrition (Per Serving)

Calories: 200

Fat: 10g

Carbohydrates: 14g

Protein 2g

The Awesome Cleanser

Serving: 2

Prep Time: 5 minutes

Ingredients:

2 grapefruits, juiced

2 lemons, juiced

Half cup alkaline water/filtered water

2 tablespoons olive oil

2 cucumbers, peeled

1 avocado, peeled and pitted

2 cloves fresh garlic

1-inch ginger

Pinch of Himalayan salt

Pinch of cayenne pepper

How To:

1. Add cucumber, ginger, avocado, grapefruit and lemon to your blender.

2. Blend until smooth.

3. Add alkaline water, spices and oil.

4. Stir well and drink chilled.

5. Enjoy!

Nutrition (Per Serving)

Calories: 200

Fat: 10g

Carbohydrates: 14g

Protein 2g

Gentle Tropical Papaya Smoothie

Serving: 2

Prep Time: 5 minutes

Ingredients:

1 papaya, cut into chunks

1 cup fat free plain yogurt

½ cup pineapple chunks

½ cup crushed ice

1 teaspoon coconut extract

1 teaspoon flaxseed

How To:

1. Add the listed ingredients to your blender and blend until smooth.

2. Serve chilled!

Nutrition (Per Serving)

Calories: 200

Fat: 10g

Carbohydrates: 14g

Protein 2g

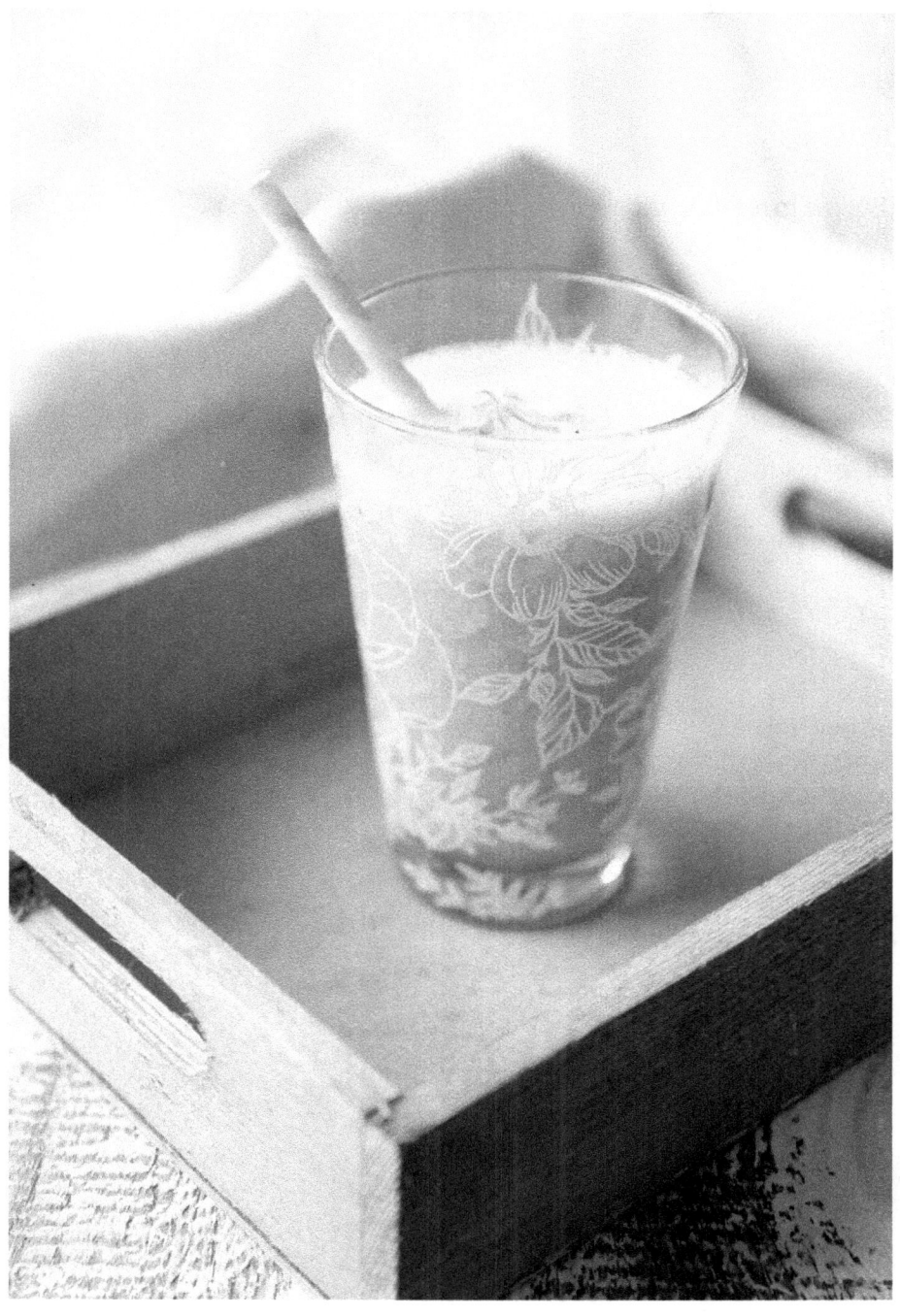

Kale and Apple Smoothie

Serving: 2

Prep Time: 5 minutes

Ingredients:

¾ of a kale, chopped, ribs and stem removed 1 small stalk celery, chopped ½ banana

½ cup apple juice

1 tablespoon lemon juice

How To:

1. Add the listed ingredients to your blender and blend until smooth.

2. Serve chilled!

Nutrition (Per Serving)

Calories: 200

Fat: 10g

Carbohydrates: 14g

Protein 2g

Mango and Lime Generous Smoothie

Serving: 2

Prep Time: 5 minutes

Ingredients:

2 tablespoons lime juice

2 cups spinach, chopped and stemmed

1 ½ cups frozen mango, cubed

1 cup green grapes

How To:

1. Add the listed ingredients to your blender and blend until smooth

2. Serve chilled!

Nutrition (Per Serving)

Calories: 200

Fat: 10g

Carbohydrates: 14g

Protein 2g

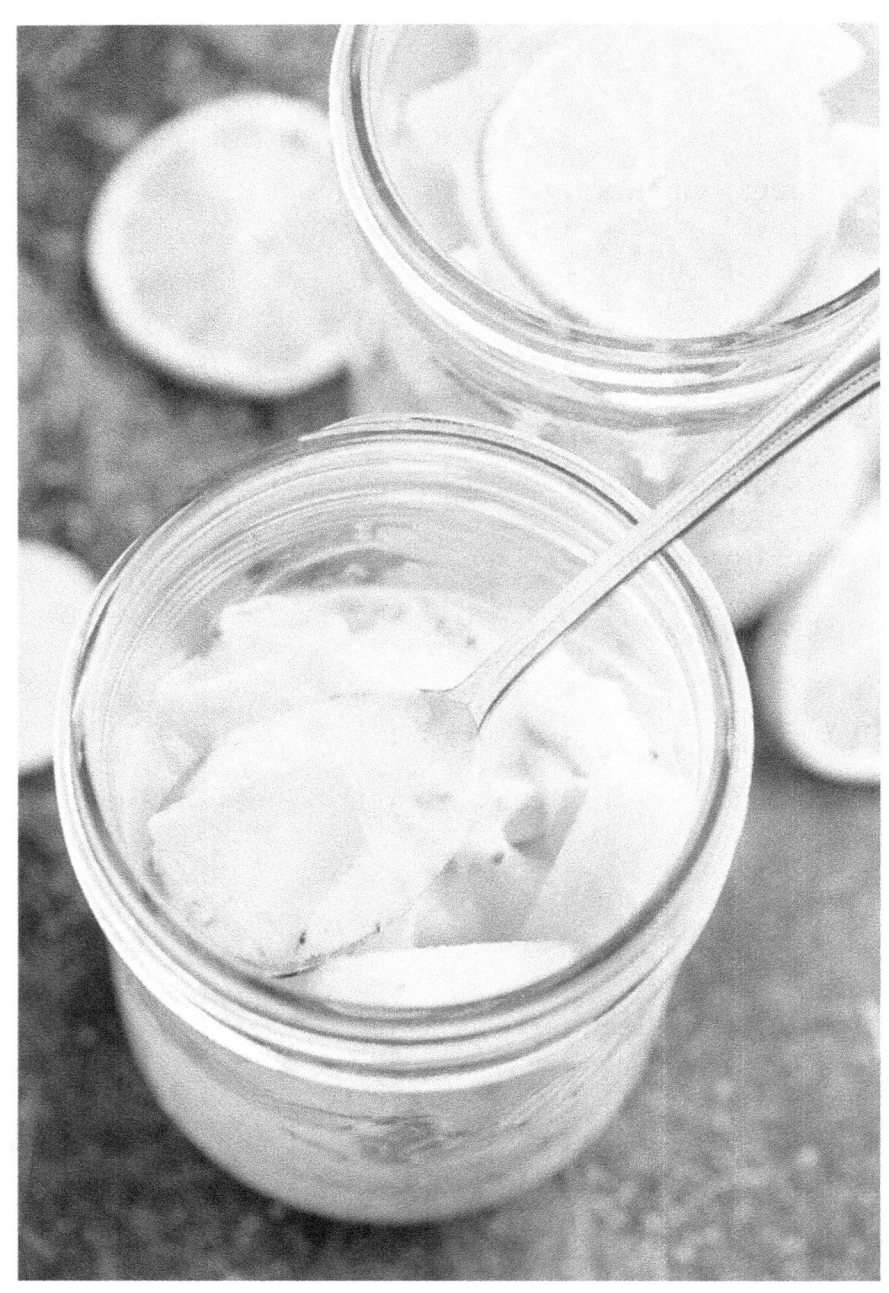

Juicy Summertime Veggies

Serving: 6

Prep Time: 10 minutes

Cooking Time: 3 hours 5 minutes

Ingredients:

1 cup grape tomatoes

2 cups okra

1 cup mushrooms

2 cups yellow bell peppers

1 ½ cup red onions

2 ½ cups zucchini

½ cup olive oil

½ cup balsamic vinegar

1 tablespoon fresh thyme, chopped

2 tablespoons fresh basil, chopped

How To:

1. Slice and chop okra, onions, tomatoes, zucchini, mushrooms.

2. Add veggies to a large container and mix.

3. Take another dish and add oil and vinegar, mix in thyme and basil.

4. Toss the veggies into the Slow Cooker and pour marinade.

5. Stir well.

6. Close lid and cook on 3 hours on HIGH, making sure to stir after every hour.

Nutrition (Per Serving)

Calories: 233

Fat: 18g

Carbohydrates: 14g

Protein: 3g

Crazy Caramelized Onion

Serving:

Prep Time: 10 minutes

Cooking Time: 9-10 hours

Ingredients:

6 onions, sliced

2 tablespoons oil

½ teaspoon salt

How To:

1. Add onions, oil and salt to your Slow Cooker.

2. Close lid and cook on LOW for 8 hours.

3. Open lid and keep simmering for 1-2 hours until any excess water has evaporated.

4. Serve and enjoy!

Nutrition (Per Serving)

Calories: 126

Fat: 15g

Carbohydrates: 15g

Protein: 2g

Kidney Beans and Cilantro

Serving: 6

Prep Time: 5 minutes

Cook Time: nil

Ingredients:

1 can (15 ounces) kidney beans, drained and rinsed ½ English cucumber, chopped

1 medium heirloom tomato, chopped

1 bunch fresh cilantro, stems removed and chopped

1 red onion, chopped

Juice of 1 large lime

3 tablespoons Dijon mustard

½ teaspoon fresh garlic paste

1 teaspoon Sumac

Salt and pepper as needed

How To:

1. Take a medium-sized bowl and add kidney beans, chopped up veggies and cilantro.

2. Take a small bowl and make the vinaigrette by adding lime juice, oil, fresh garlic, pepper, mustard and Sumac.

3. Pour the vinaigrette over the salad and give it a gentle stir.

4. Add some salt and pepper.

5. Cover and allow to chill for half an hour.

6. Serve!

Nutrition (Per Serving)

Calories: 74

Fat: 0.7g

Carbohydrates: 16g

Protein: 21g

Broccoli Crunchies

Serving: 4

Prep Time: 10 minutes

Cooking Time: 3 hours

Ingredients:

2 cups broccoli florets

2 ounces cream of celery soup

2 tablespoons cheddar cheese, shredded

1 small yellow onion, chopped

¼ teaspoon Worcestershire sauce

Salt and pepper as needed

½ tablespoon butter

How To:

1. Add broccoli, cream, cheese, onion, cheddar to Slow Cooker.

2. Stir and season with salt and pepper.

3. Place lid and cook on LOW for 3 hours.

4. Serve and enjoy!

Nutrition (Per Serving)

Calories: 162

Fat: 11g

Carbohydrates: 11g

Protein: 5g

Ultimate Buffalo Cashews

Serving: 4

Prep Time: 10 minutes

Cook Time: 55 minutes

Ingredients:

2 cups raw cashews

¾ cup red hot sauce

1/3 cup avocado oil

½ teaspoon garlic powder

¼ teaspoon turmeric

How To:

1.   Take a bowl, mix the wet ingredients in a bowl and stir in seasoning.

2.   Add cashews to the bowl and mix.

3.   Soak cashews in hot sauce mix for 2-4 hours.

4.   Pre-heat your oven to 325 degrees F.

5. Spread cashews onto baking sheet.

6. Bake for 35-55 minutes, turning after every 10-15 minutes.

7. Let them cool and serve!

Nutrition (Per Serving)

Calories: 268

Fat: 16g

Carbohydrates: 20g

Protein: 14g

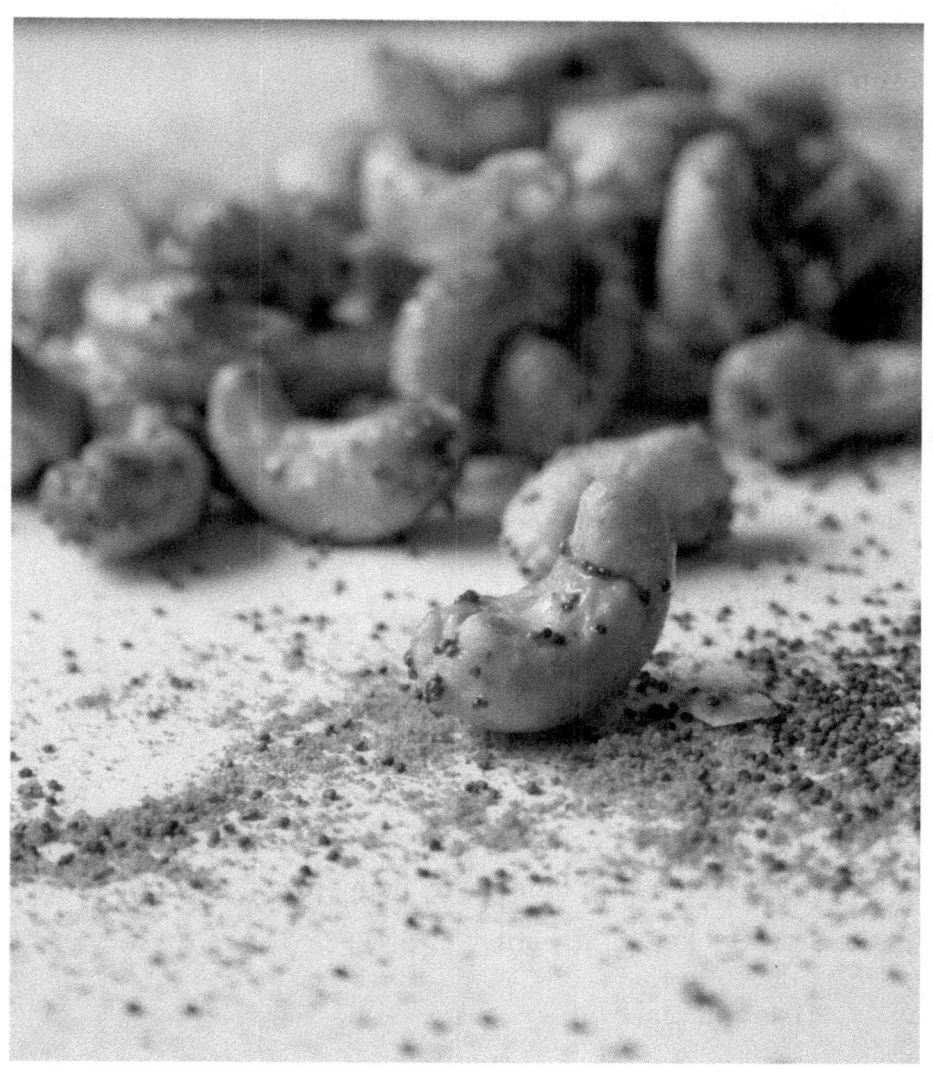

A Green Bean Mixture

Serving: 2

Prep Time: 10 minutes

Cooking Time: 2 hours

Ingredients:

4 cups green beans, trimmed

2 tablespoons butter, melted

1 tablespoon date paste

Salt and pepper as needed

¼ teaspoon coconut aminos

How To:

1. Add green beans, date paste, pepper, salt, coconut aminos to the Slow Cooker, gently stir.
2. Toss and place lid.
3. Cook on LOW for 2 hours.
4. Serve and enjoy!

Nutrition (Per Serving)

Calories: 236

Fat: 6g

Carbohydrates: 10g

Protein: 6g

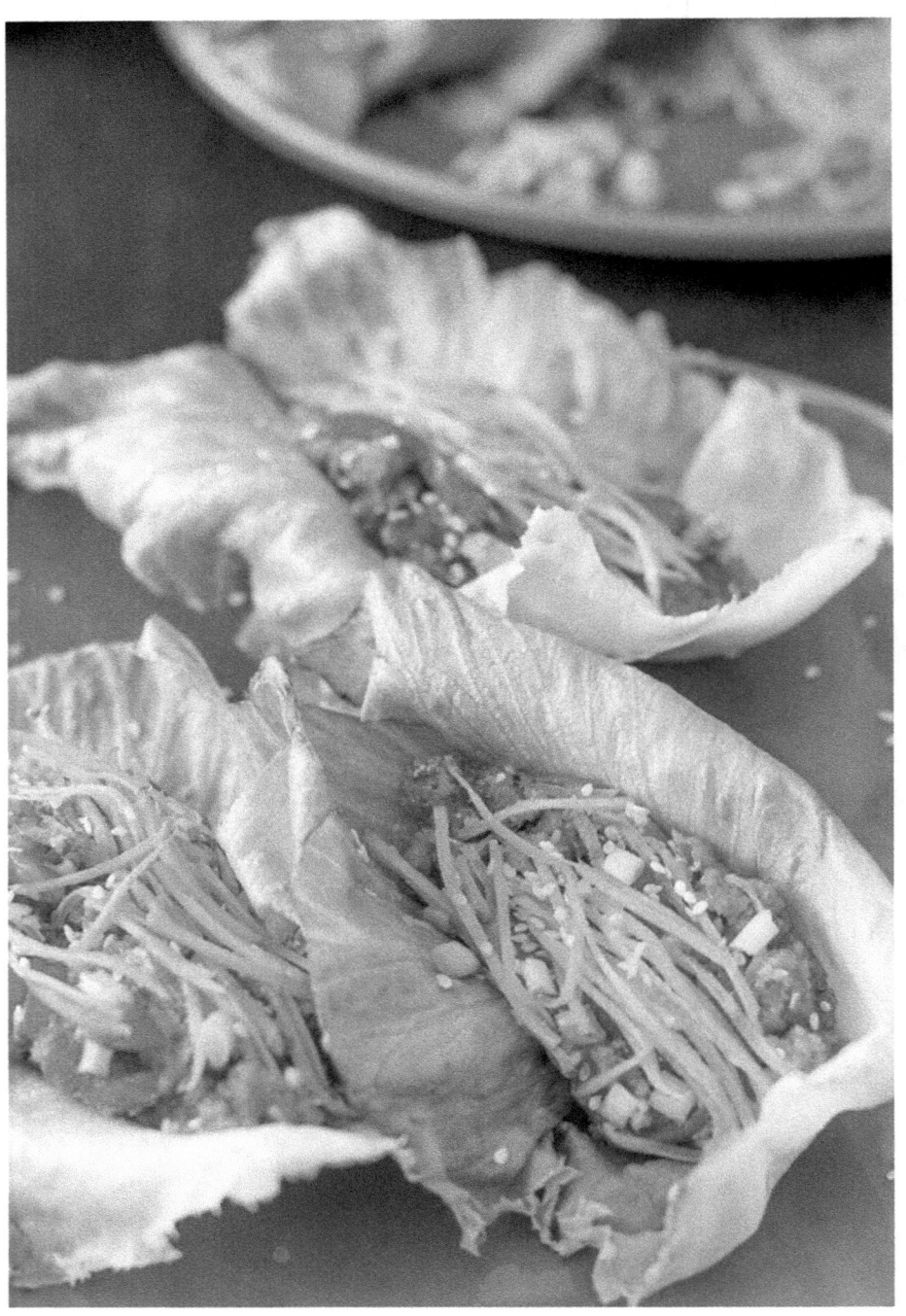

www.ingramcontent.com/pod-product-compliance
Lightning Source LLC
Chambersburg PA
CBHW071109030426
42336CB00013BA/2018